"Nobody lives forever, we just chug along, until the track runs out. But, we might be able to slow down that train, and sometimes we can add some track."

— Lance Hodge

5-Minute CPR:
A Paramedic's Guide to Simple CPR

Copyright Lance Hodge, 2017

ISBN 13: 978-1547285488

Printed in the United States of America

Updated: 2/20

5-Minute CPR:
A Paramedic's Guide to Simple CPR

By Lance Hodge, Paramedic

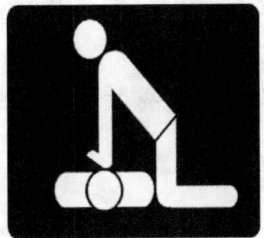

This book is about being *prepared to act* in a medical emergency where CPR is needed; I'll also talk briefly about the *basics* of first aid.

The book is titled "5-Minute CPR" because learning "Hands Only" CPR is quick and could be done in five minutes.

I'm a Paramedic. I worked for the *Los Angeles City Fire Department* for more than a decade. I hurt my back carrying a man down a flight of stairs and was forced to retire. I now teach a college EMT course. During my time as an active Paramedic I handled at least 15,000 9-1-1 calls, of all the sorts of things you'd imagine a Paramedic in a big city might encounter. Hundreds of those calls involved cardiac issues, and cardiac arrest. We saved some of those people, but not nearly enough. Part of the problem, in not being able to save more people, is a combination of two main factors. One, bystanders usually weren't doing CPR when we arrived, or if they were, it was being done incorrectly and was not very effective. The second problem, and that will be discussed later in this book, is that the *defibrillator* got to the patient too late. We tried, but despite the most efficient EMS system's efforts, if the rescuers arrive 7, 8, or more minutes after the cardiac arrest has occurred (and normal response times are often longer) the chance that the defibrillation will work to bring about an effective heart rhythm, goes *way* down. We'll discuss just what *defibrillation* means as we continue.

~

In the event of a medical emergency, it is not knowing what to do that most often creates panic in people, mistaken intervention, and ultimately regret that they should have done more. *We need to know what to do!*

CPR is often misrepresented, as a *life-saving* technique; although it *is* that, *sometimes*, most often despite our best efforts the person will not survive, even with the intervention of proper CPR. *CPR alone isn't enough.* There is no guarantee with CPR, but it offers one of the best chances for the bystander to help, and the *only* chance before advanced medical care arrives. (Unless a defibrillator is available on site.)

This book is simple, and short, for a reason. We all know we could take a CPR class, but most of us don't. It can be expensive, and it takes time, often several hours.

Some of us have learned CPR in the past, but we forgot a lot of it. Learning CPR can be somewhat overwhelming; there's adult CPR, child CPR, infant CPR, and choking procedures for each, and differences depending on if they are responsive or unresponsive with an airway obstruction. The differences between adult, child and infant procedures can be confusing. Every few years the *American Heart Association®* and *American Red Cross®* change a few things, making even those who have been trained doubt if they know what the most current procedure is. Doubt often results in inaction, people simply call 9-1-1 and don't step in to help.

Calling 9-1-1. We'll discuss this again later; calling 9-1-1 is VITAL, but it isn't enough, rescuers often won't get there soon enough to revive the person in cardiac arrest. If EMT's or Paramedics don't arrive in just a *few minutes*, the chances go WAY down that their intervention will be successful. ***The AED (defibrillator) MUST be used in the first few minutes in cardiac arrest or it may not work.***

EMT's and Paramedics. Generally, firefighters are often trained as EMT's (Emergency Medical Technicians) and sometimes also as Paramedics. Firefighters usually have defibrillators on their apparatus, just like ambulances. Paramedics do everything an EMT can do but also have more training in some special techniques, including EKG interpretation, inserting advanced airways (Endotracheal tubes) and starting IV's. They also have many medications they can administer, especially *cardiac* related medications. A Paramedic unit is basically a *mobile Emergency Room* when it comes to the immediate treatment of a person in cardiac arrest. *Cardiac arrest* means the heart has stopped beating, and when that happens breathing also stops. Often it is a *heart attack* that damages the heart and causes *cardiac arrest* by causing the heart to begin to quiver (ventricular fibrillation) instead of beating. A heart attack can be big or small, the victim may be awake during it or become unconscious or the heart can stop completely, causing *Cardiac arrest*. A *heart attack* is not the only cause of *cardiac arrest*, drugs may cause it, breathing difficulties may cause it, even electrocution and many other reasons.

Lay people **(the general public)** rarely have an opportunity to use their CPR skills after completing their CPR class, (EMT's and Paramedics get a LOT of practice) and after a short time those people who took a CPR class become less confident that they will remember what to do if an emergency occurs.

This book will concentrate on two main points, to hopefully deal with the issue of *confusion* and *forgetting*. First, we'll keep it *simple*. We'll concentrate on **Adult CPR**. That is the most likely life-threatening cardiac issue you would encounter where CPR is needed. Children and infants are much more likely to have some respiratory emergency occur, which *could* then lead to cardiac arrest, and that does require a bit more study involving obstructed airways and those more confusing child and infant procedural differences. It is advised that you take a complete CPR course, to cover all these various issues. This book will concentrate on *Adult Hands Only CPR*; that should help to avoid *confusion*. Second, this is a *short* book, you can read the whole thing in one sitting, in a short amount of time. That should help with *forgetting* what you've learned, since you can easily read the book again from time to time, to keep this information fresh in your mind.

Cardio Pulmonary Resuscitation is all about the *heart* and the *lungs*. We push on the chest to cause blood to flow, and if breaths are given, we add some oxygen to the blood stream… but. "Hands Only" CPR is what this book will cover. With *Hands Only* CPR we do **NOT** give breaths. That makes things easier, and more likely that you might do CPR to a stranger. The good news is that pushing on the chest, doing our CPR chest compressions, *also* pushes air in and out of the lungs. So, we don't NEED to give breaths to the victim, it happens automatically! Think of how slow and shallow you might be breathing while you sleep, that's plenty of oxygen to keep you alive, we don't need much; but if we don't get it, if we just lay there, with no heartbeat and no breathing, we'll die in just a few minutes. *Hands Only CPR* will provide enough oxygen, without giving them breaths!

Time is the enemy. The brain is *very* delicate when it comes to being deprived of oxygen. Brain cells die within 4-6 minutes without proper oxygenation. It will take rescuers longer than 4-6 minutes to arrive and begin their treatment. We must act, and we must call 9-1-1 *immediately* then begin CPR and *continue CPR* until help arrives and takes over! Don't stop!

Denial: People having a heart attack often *deny* there is a real problem and blame how they are feeling on something else; something they ate, being tired, the heat, the humidity, working too hard, etc… the list is long and it is the reason that so many people having a heart attack don't call 9-1-1 right away, they stay home too long, they allow the heart attack to get worse, and ultimately many will die who may have been able to be saved. If someone looks or feels awful (pale, sweaty, short of breath, nauseated, chest/jaw/arm pain, a skipping pulse) don't let them blame it on something else and stay home, **CALL 9-1-1** whether they want you to or not! *Call right away and don't wait!* When you aren't sure if you should call 9-1-1 or not, **CALL 9-1-1**.

It's up to you! CPR is our attempt to circulate oxygenated blood to the brain and other organs. CPR may buy us some time. If we initiate CPR, we might extend that inevitable death of brain cells beyond those 4-6 minutes, so that the victim is more viable to resuscitation when those rescuers arrive. The other factor, and it is the *most important* key to saving the life of someone in cardiac arrest, is the *defibrillator*. (*Costco* sells them!)

The defibrillator. First, cardiac arrest means that the heart has ceased a functional heartbeat, most often the heart is in *Ventricular Fibrillation*, meaning it is simply quivering, and not pumping blood. A "**Defibrillator**" shocks the heart, overwhelming all electrical activity, and essentially *stops* the heart completely, getting rid of Ventricular Fibrillation. That doesn't sound good, but once the fibrillation is stopped it is hoped that the heart is not too damaged and that the pacemaker cells within the heart will *recharge* and that a viable heartbeat will spontaneously begin. That's what the defibrillator does. An "AED" is a mostly automatic, simple *defibrillator*, most often used by EMT's or by lay-rescuers. A more complicated *manual* defibrillator, which has other functions, including an EKG screen to *see* the heart rhythm, will defibrillate just like an AED and is often used by Paramedics, who have more training than EMT's. The manual defibrillator, or the AED (Automated External Defibrillator) will both do the same thing for defibrillation of ventricular fibrillation.

9-1-1 gets us the defibrillator. For every minute that passes before defibrillation occurs there is a 10% less chance that the defibrillator will reverse the fibrillation. After eight minutes, as an example, there is an 80% chance that the defibrillation attempts will fail. We must get a defibrillator to the victim *quickly* if they are to have the best chance of being revived. **<u>If you are somewhere that has an AED available, you can use it!</u>** If the person has no pulse and no breathing, we should attach the AED; they are simple, the patches that go on the chest have pictures on them, of where they should be placed. Turn on the machine and it will talk you through each step. It's easy, and you're allowed to use it! The AED is THE most important tool to save a person in cardiac arrest. In an emergency ask if there is an AED on scene, have someone get it, now.

Death. When the heart stops beating, breathing stops. No heartbeat and no breathing is defined as "death." People who die, usually stay dead. CPR along with rapid defibrillation gives the victim the best chance, and some people *will* be revived. If the brain has not been too damaged, the person may make a full, or nearly full, recovery. If the cardiac arrest has been caused by a significant "heart attack" it is possible that none of our efforts, CPR nor defibrillation, will save them. The heart may have suffered too much damage to function again.

A "heart attack" means death of some heart muscle. We don't know if someone has had a "heart attack" until tests are done at the hospital. Other things might cause the heart to stop beating properly; medications, drugs, respiratory problems, electric shock, to name a few. Remember, *cardiac arrest* means the heart and breathing has stopped, but that does not always mean a "Heart Attack" has occurred. ***Regardless of what has caused the condition the person needs to get to the hospital right now!***

Not breathing. If a person's heart is still beating (they have a pulse) but they have stopped breathing, that is called "respiratory arrest." *Michael Jackson* and *Prince* are two high-profile examples. Medications or other drugs depressed their breathing until it stopped, and after a few minutes of no breathing the heart will stop beating and begin to *fibrillate* (quiver and not pump) and the person will end up in cardiac arrest. If quick CPR and defibrillation does not occur, the person will die. In ***Respiratory Arrest*** the person has a pulse and only needs breaths to be given, <u>not</u> CPR chest compressions. If we aren't **SURE** they are breathing or not, or if the breathing is very weak and irregular, we SHOULD DO CPR.

CPR chest compressions will move air in and out of the lungs with each compression along with circulating blood to the brain.

Other stuff. There's a bunch of other things we could talk about, but we're keeping it simple here. Again, it's recommended that you take the time to take a CPR course, even a first aid course, there's a lot more to learn.

Checking the pulse. So far, we haven't talked much about checking the victim's pulse. Some studies have shown that people aren't very good at determining whether a person has a pulse or not. Elsewhere in this book, checking the pulse will be discussed as one of the steps. Generally, in the most basic CPR classes, such as "Hands Only" CPR, the pulse is **not** checked, but is replaced by checking the person for any signs of movement or breathing. If they appear lifeless, CPR is begun. If you **do** check a pulse, and they *definitely* have one, CPR is *not* needed. If you aren't **SURE** there is or isn't a pulse, or if you're not **SURE** the person is breathing, act as if there is no pulse or breathing, and **begin CPR.**

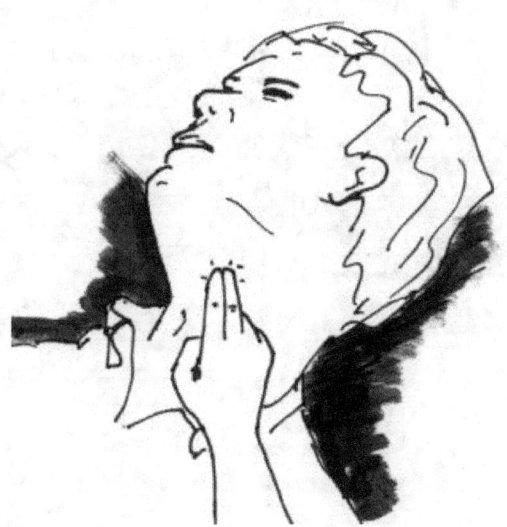

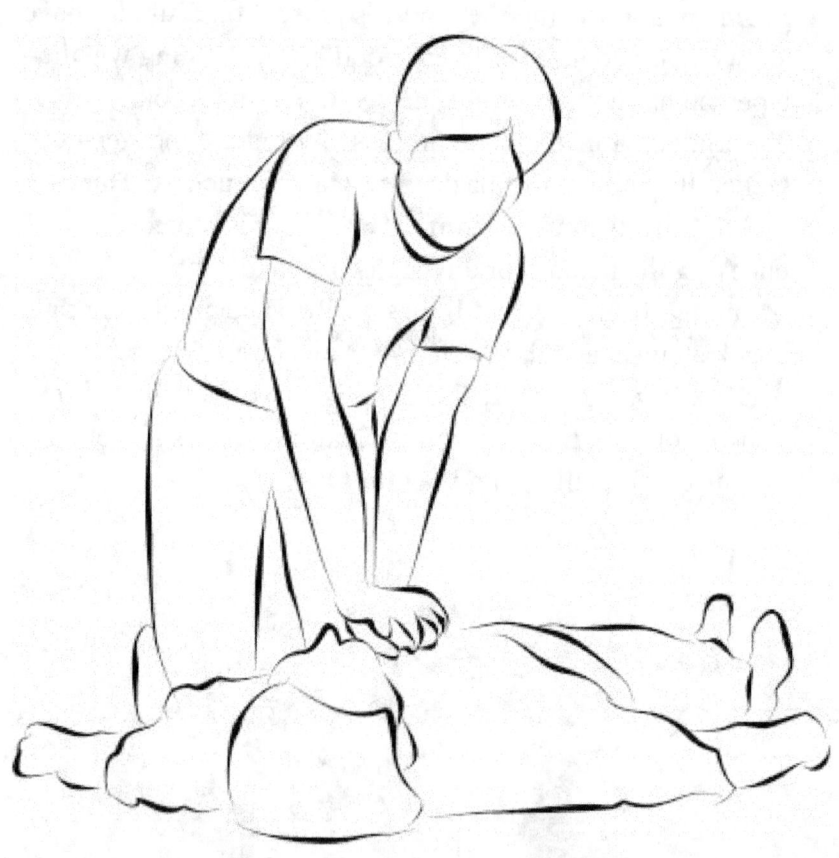

HANDS ONLY CPR.

We just push on the chest, that's it!

Simplicity has its advantages; there's less to remember.

We're more likely to DO CPR and less likely to panic if we believe we know what to do. We'll feel confident that we have done everything we could, when what we do is simple, and we know we've done it correctly.

Hands Only CPR

is simple.

1

We shout, "Are you OK!" at the person. We should **tap their shoulder <u>firmly</u>**. If they respond in any way, they are alive, and don't need CPR. (That's where some first aid training would be nice, there's some other things we might want to do)

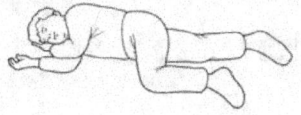

If they didn't respond, we look at them carefully, for about **five seconds**, for any sign of movement, sound, or breathing. If they are responding in any way, they are alive, and don't need CPR.

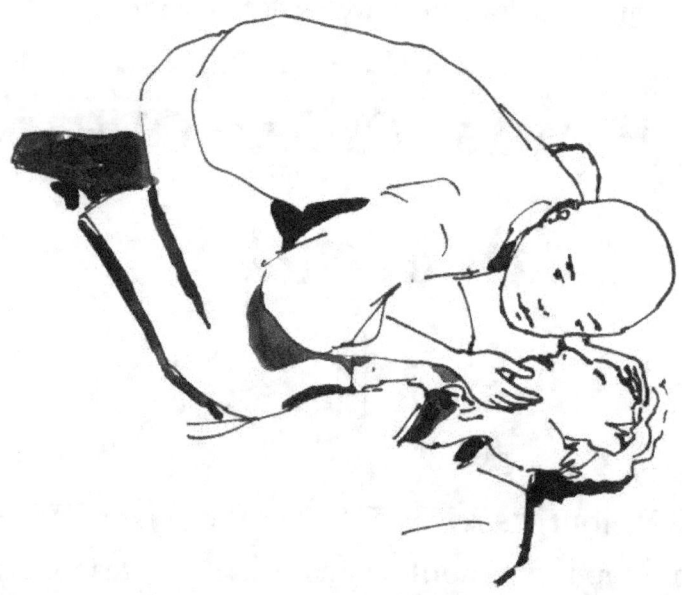

This photo shows the person using the 'head-tilt chin-lift' to open the airway. Push down on the forehead and pull up on the chin to tilt the head back, which moves the tongue up, to help open the airway.

3

If there was no response to your shout or shoulder tap, and no sign of movement or breathing after checking for five seconds, they need CPR.

Start chest compressions.

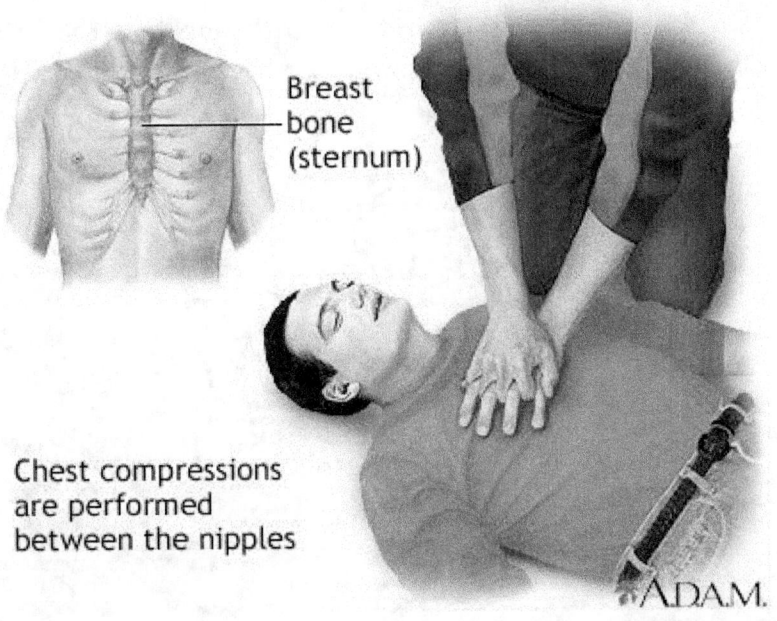

Breast bone (sternum)

Chest compressions are performed between the nipples

A.D.A.M.

The center of the heel of one hand is placed on the sternum, and centered at an imaginary nipple line, with the other hand on top of the first, fingers are interlaced and pulled up off the chest.

→ We push down at least 2 inches deep, which is probably *harder* than you think you should push.

→ We push at a rate of 100 times per minute, which is the beat of the *Bee Gees* song *"Stayin Alive."*

And we keep going...

We keep pushing at this rate, and that depth, and we keep going until help arrives and takes over.

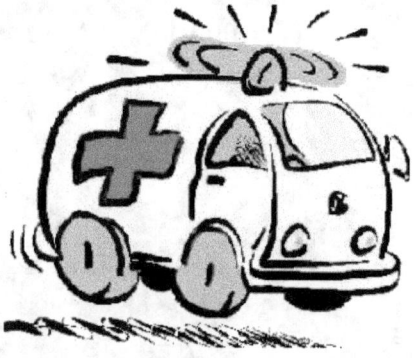

Note:

Make sure your hand comes up completely after each push down on the chest, leaving no pressure on the chest, this is called "Full chest recoil" and will make your CPR even more effective.

That was it.

Hands Only CPR is that simple.

~

→ Shout "Are you OK?" and tap their shoulder firmly for several seconds. *Call 9-1-1!*

→ Check for any sign of movement or breathing for 5 seconds, if none, start chest compressions.

→ Push hard and fast, at least 2 inches deep, at a rate of 100 times per minute.

Keep going... help is on the way.

You should be able to find short CPR videos online to further clarify and demonstrate proper hand placement on the chest. Also, re-read this book frequently, so that you don't forget these steps and the other information in this book. Tell your friends, spread the word!

Page 19, 20, and 21 talks about some things you would learn in a more advanced CPR course, such as child and infant CPR and Choking. These things are also simple but can lead to confusion over time.   Information like this is easily forgotten unless the skills are practiced frequently.

Continuing reading but remember that this additional information about CPR and Choking may create confusion, and you may forget much of it. <u>Frequent study of this book and all this information will help to ensure that you know what to do if an emergency situation occurs</u>.

Concentrate on *Hands Only CPR*. Adult cardiac arrest is the most common life-threatening event you might expect to encounter.

If you can afford it, keep an AED in the home!

More information. This is NOT meant to be complete or to replace a CPR course but is some additional information in case you're interested. This guide goes beyond "Hands Only" CPR, adding some items normally included in a more advanced CPR class.

~

"5-MINUTE CPR"
A Paramedic's Guide to Simple CPR

By Lance Hodge, Paramedic, *Former L.A. City Fire Dept. Paramedic, College EMT Instructor*

These instructions may include breaths, which could be vital in the event of a breathing emergency, especially in children and infants. **You may use "Hands Only" CPR with NO breaths for unresponsive adults.**

<u>Note</u>: *This is a modified 'summary' of key points. Study a CPR textbook for more details and take a CPR class to practice these skills.*

<u>Note</u>: *When giving breaths, use an approved barrier device to avoid contact with bodily fluids.*

<u>Infant</u>: newborn to one year old ♦ <u>Child</u>: 1 to adolescent (puberty)

<u>Adult</u>: Adolescent and older

►**First**, call, or have someone else **call 9-1-1**

(<u>You must get a *defibrillator* to the patient as soon as possible</u>! For every minute that passes, there is a 10% LESS chance that the defibrillator will work to convert the heart back to a functioning heartbeat. Time is critical! **We must get an AED quickly!**)

▲ *(If there is the likelihood of serious neck or back injury, be careful not to move the neck and spine, NO head tilt!)*

►Check for responsiveness **(Tap & Shout)**

FIRMLY tap the shoulder for several seconds, shout, **"Are you OK?"**

If there is no response, move to the next step. (►Open the airway)

If they **do** respond and seem to be breathing ok, place them on their side and wait for help. If the person is **awake** *and* severely choking (adult or child), reach around, place your fist 'just' above belly button, place other fist on top of first, give five inward and upward *firm* thrusts (Heimlich Maneuver) and repeat until the object is expelled. For *awake* and severely choking ***infants***, give 5 firm back slaps (between shoulder blades), followed by 5 chest compressions (just like in CPR), repeat until the airway is open.

If the choking person becomes <u>unresponsive</u>, begin CPR chest compressions 30:2, which may dislodge the object; and check the mouth for any object before giving breaths.

►**Open the airway** with a "Head Tilt, Chin Lift" maneuver *(Push down on forehead, pull up under chin)*

►**Check for breathing** *and* **pulse**, for 5 seconds. If no breathing and no pulse, start CPR chest compressions. If they <u>have a pulse</u>, but are <u>not breathing</u>, give a breath *only*, every 3-5 seconds; **no** compressions if there is a pulse.

▲ If breaths do not go in **(if chest does not rise)**, this indicates an airway obstruction; **begin CPR chest compressions**, this may dislodge the object.

▲ **When dealing with choking (obstructed airway) Check the mouth after 30 chest compressions** *before* attempting to give a breath. Remove any object that you can **SEE**, by using a *hooking motion* deeply into the mouth, from the cheek first to avoid pushing the object deeper.

▲ **Try to give two breaths** again. **If they do not go in, continue CPR chest compressions,** checking the mouth each time for an object before attempting to give a breath. Repeat until the airway is clear.

►**If two breaths go in, <u>check the neck for a pulse</u>** *(check pulse in upper arm of infants, under the bicep).* Take 5 seconds to feel for a pulse. <u>**If you aren't SURE there is a pulse, start CPR chest compressions**</u>.

▲ **If they have a pulse, make sure they are breathing** at least once every five seconds, if they *have a pulse* and are *not* breathing, give them a breath every five seconds *(Rescue Breathing), every 3 seconds for children and infants. (Use a barrier device when giving mouth-to-mouth breathing)* **If they have a pulse and are breathing, but are unresponsive**, *call 9-1-1, place them on their side, check pulse and breathing every few minutes.*

►**If they do not have a pulse, begin chest compressions**. Place the heel of one hand on the middle of the sternum, at the nipple line, place other hand on top of first *(Use one or two hands for Children)* Push down *at least* 2 inches *(for adults)* 2 inches for children, and 1 ½ inches for infants, all at a rate of 100/min. (the beat of the *Bee Gees* song, "Stayin Alive") Give 30 compressions, and then give 2 breaths. Repeat. **Do not stop** to reassess, *unless* you see signs of life, movement, or breathing. Continue CPR, 30 compressions then 2 breaths, until help arrives. *(Ensure that you allow the chest to fully recoil, come all the way UP, after each chest compression).*

Infant CPR: (Newborn to 1-year-old) Use the tips of two fingers on the middle of the chest, 'just' *below* an imaginary line between the nipples. Push down 1 ½ inches, at a rate of 100/min.

Do 30 compressions, then give 2 breaths. Repeat. **Do not stop**. *Allow full chest recoil.*

21

KEEP TRYING! Choking procedures may not be effective at first. Keep trying!

Don't expect CPR to revive the person, they need EMTs or Paramedics with a defibrillator and medications. Keep doing CPR!

Call 9-1-1 FIRST!

SOME FIRST AID BASICS:

Try not to get another person's blood or bodily fluids on you. Use latex gloves when possible.

Shock:

Being "In shock" means you aren't getting proper blood flow to all the parts of your body, usually causing dizziness, paleness, sweatiness, fainting, nausea or vomiting, low blood pressure, and a fast pulse. There are many possible causes. Call 9-1-1. The person should be put in "shock position" lying on their back with their legs somewhat elevated. If they are confused or unresponsive, place them on their *side*; in case they vomit, they'll be less likely to choke.

Note: If some medical problem, any medical problem, which may include possible heart attack, causes the person to appear "shocky" lie them down. (*Exception: If the person is having trouble breathing, or signs of a stroke, try to keep them sitting up, don't lay them down.*)

Note: If the person having trouble breathing faints, *then* lay them down and treat for shock.

Bleeding:

Severe, life-threatening bleeding is usually easily controlled with firm direct pressure on the area. Use your gloved hand or fingers directly on the area or place a cloth or napkin on the area and then apply firm pressure on top of it. Don't release the pressure! Don't remove the dressing you placed on it to 'check it.' Call 9-1-1 or see a doctor.

Trauma:

Some violent force, a fall, car accident, broken bone, etc. Be careful not to move, bend, or twist the victim, in case they have a neck/spine injury. Keep them still, call 9-1-1. If you must move them for safety reasons try to keep their body in line, not twisted; dragging them by their feet, or pulling their clothes near the feet or shoulders may help to keep them more aligned.

Burns:

Cool the area with cool water, to stop the burning process. Do not apply ointments to severe burns. Call 9-1-1 or see a doctor.

Trouble breathing:

Call 9-1-1. Keep them sitting up, if they faint, lay them down. Tilt the head back to open the airway.

Impaled object:

Something stuck into the body. Call 9-1-1. Don't remove the object, unless you *must* remove it to do CPR or another life-saving procedure.

Stroke:

A bleed or blood clot in the brain. May have headache, one-sided weakness or paralysis, slurred speech, blurred vision, confusion. Blood pressure is often high, try to keep victim sitting up, unless they faint, then lay them down. Call 9-1-1.

Heart attack:

Chest pain, arm or jaw pain, pale, sweaty, dizzy, nausea/vomiting. Treat for shock, call 9-1-1.

Drug or alcohol overdose, or unconscious:

Lay them on their side, to keep them from choking if they vomit. Call 9-1-1. *(Page 13 has a drawing of "Recovery position" which is how you place them securely on their side)*

Note:
When in doubt, and something seems wrong, call 9-1-1. Don't delay, call 9-1-1.

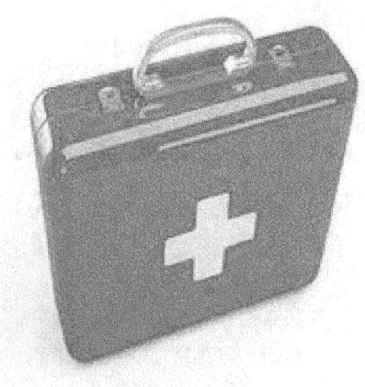

Other books by Lance Hodge:

*Available at **Amazon.com**, Booksamillion.com,*

Barnes & Noble, and other fine booksellers.

~

<u>Kids:</u>

A Kid's Book of First Aid
> https://www.createspace.com/5123412

A Kid's Book of First Aid 2
> https://www.createspace.com/6681283

~

Approach your church, school, or other group about starting a program to teach kids the basics of first aid, using the books listed above just for kids!

~

You could save a life!

Share this book with friends and family, better yet, buy them their own book! Makes a great gift!

www.ingramcontent.com/pod-product-compliance
Lightning Source LLC
Chambersburg PA
CBHW061951280526
45787CB00004B/1811